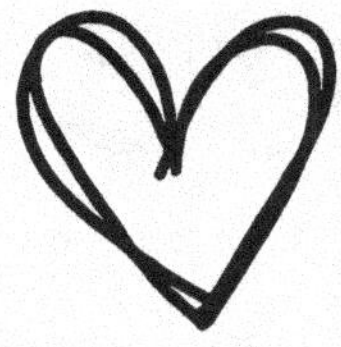

To Sandra, my strength and my inspiration.

Each day by your side is a gift, and the love we share drives me to be better every moment. Your strength, your beauty, and the partnership we've built make our journey even more extraordinary. I'm deeply grateful to you, my love, for being the foundation of our marriage and for walking with me through this life of growth, love, and evolution.

With all my love,
Nader

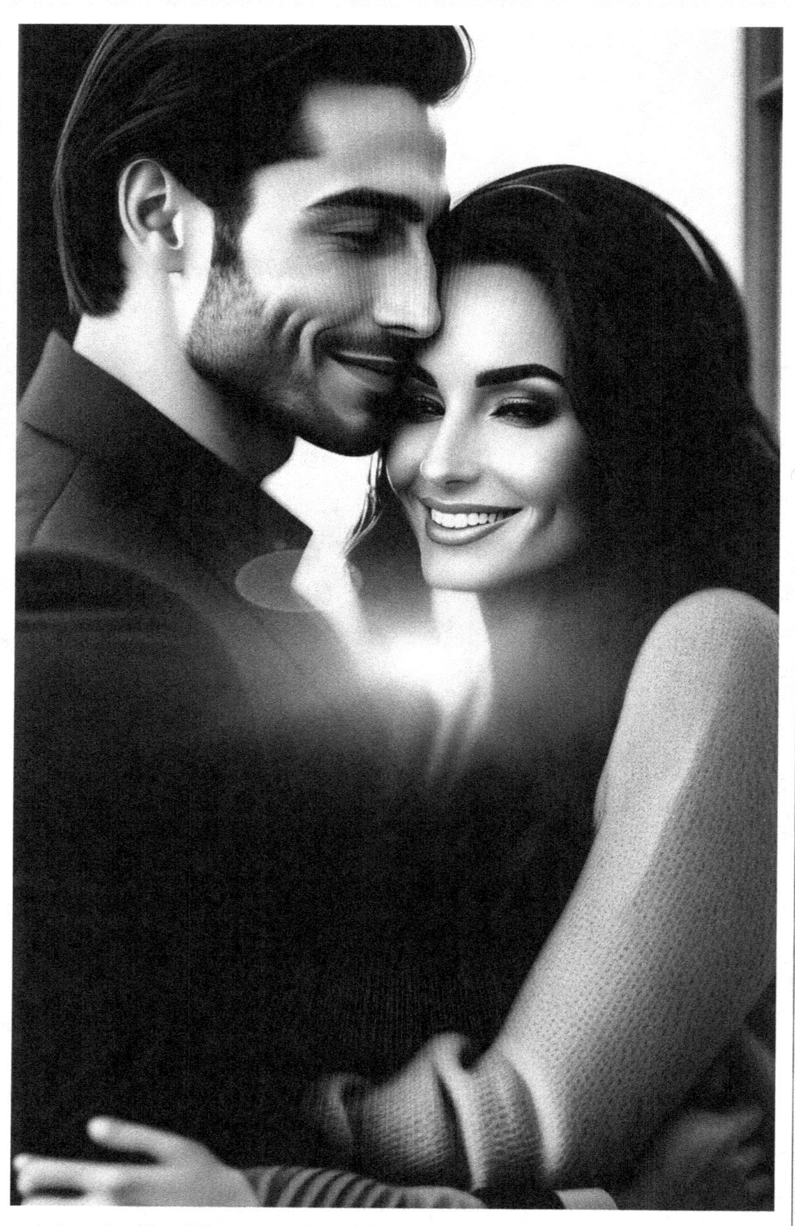

Introduction

This e-book aims at men seeking to create more self-awareness, confidence, and wisdom to achieve a healthy marriage.

Marriage is one of life's most meaningful experiences, and it can also be challenging.

To build a healthy and satisfying relationship, developing emotional and psychological skills, such as self-awareness, empathy, gratitude, and forgiveness is important.

In this e-book, we'll provide you with practical tips and exercises to help you develop that strong character within you.

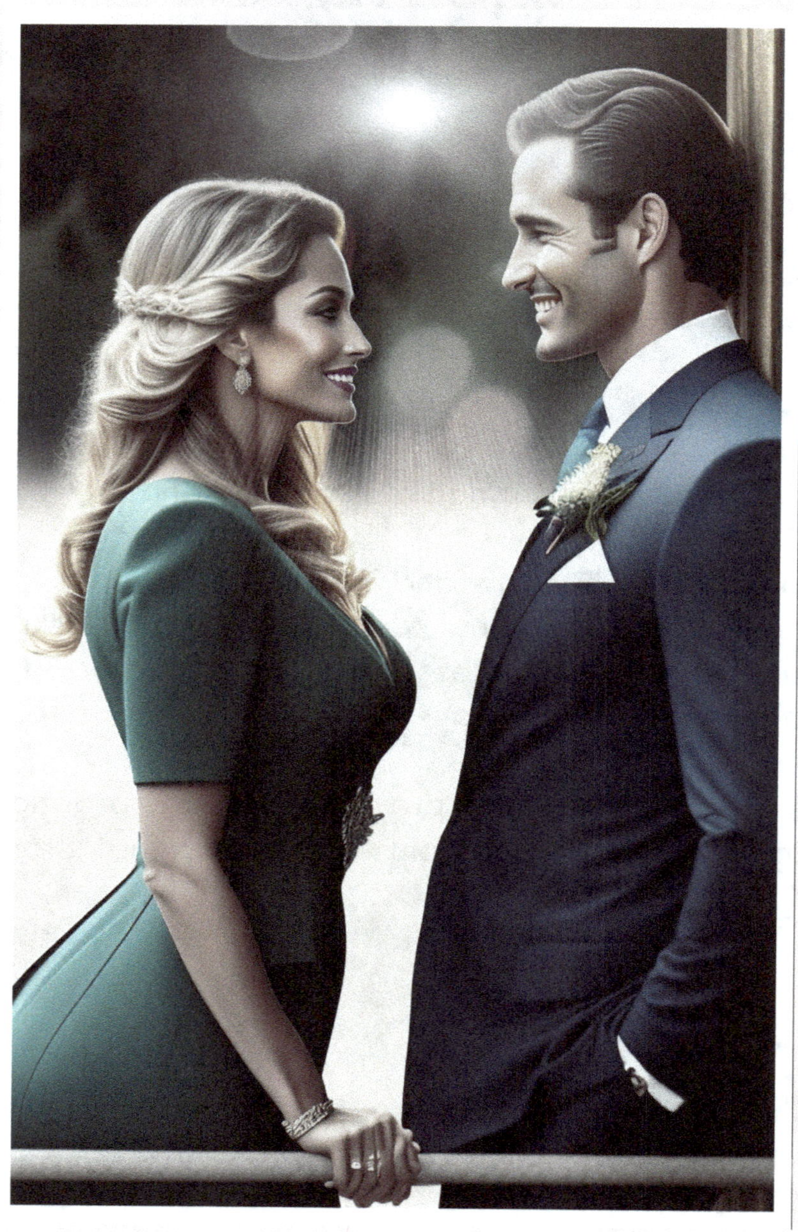

Chapter 1

Self-knowledge and self-esteem

A healthy marriage starts with a healthy relationship with yourself. Self-knowledge and self-esteem are fundamental for the development of a sense of identity, self-confidence, and self-respect, essential for building a loving and satisfying relationship.

Self-awareness is the key to creating a healthy and meaningful relationship. When you get to know yourself better, you can understand your needs, desires, and limitations and communicate them more clearly to your partner. In this chapter, we'll talk about the importance of self-awareness and self-esteem and provide tips and exercises to help you develop these skills.

The importance of self-knowledge and self-esteem for a healthy marriage

Self-knowledge is the ability to understand your thoughts, emotions, values, and behaviors. When you know yourself well, you can make more conscious decisions and be more clear about your needs, desires, and limitations. This allows you to communicate more effectively with your partner, resolve conflicts more constructively, and set healthy boundaries in your relationship.

Self-esteem is the assessment you make of yourself. When you have positive self-esteem, you are better able to love and respect yourself, which leads to healthier relationships. Also, when you feel good about yourself, you are better able to relate to others positively and constructively.

Tips and exercises to develop self-knowledge and self-esteem:

- **Practice self-reflection:** It can be beneficial to take a moment to examine your thoughts, feelings, emotions, and actions. Consider writing down your observations and taking time to contemplate them.

- **Make a list of your values:** Identify the values that are important to you and how they influence your decisions and actions.

- **Practice acceptance:** learn to accept yourself, with all your faults and imperfections. Remember that we all make mistakes and that this is all part of the learning and growing process.

- **Take care:** Take care of your physical and mental health. Practice physical exercises, sleep well, have a healthy diet, and seek activities that bring you joy and satisfaction.

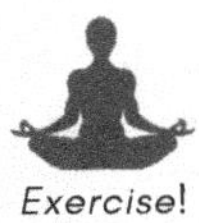

Exercise!

- **Seek Professional Help:** If you are having trouble developing self-awareness and self-esteem, consider seeking help from a mental health professional.

By developing self-awareness and self-esteem, you will be building a strong foundation for a healthy marriage.

Remember, this is an ongoing process that takes practice and dedication, but the benefits are priceless.

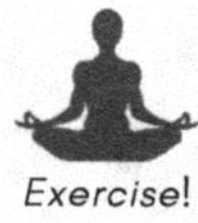

Exercise!

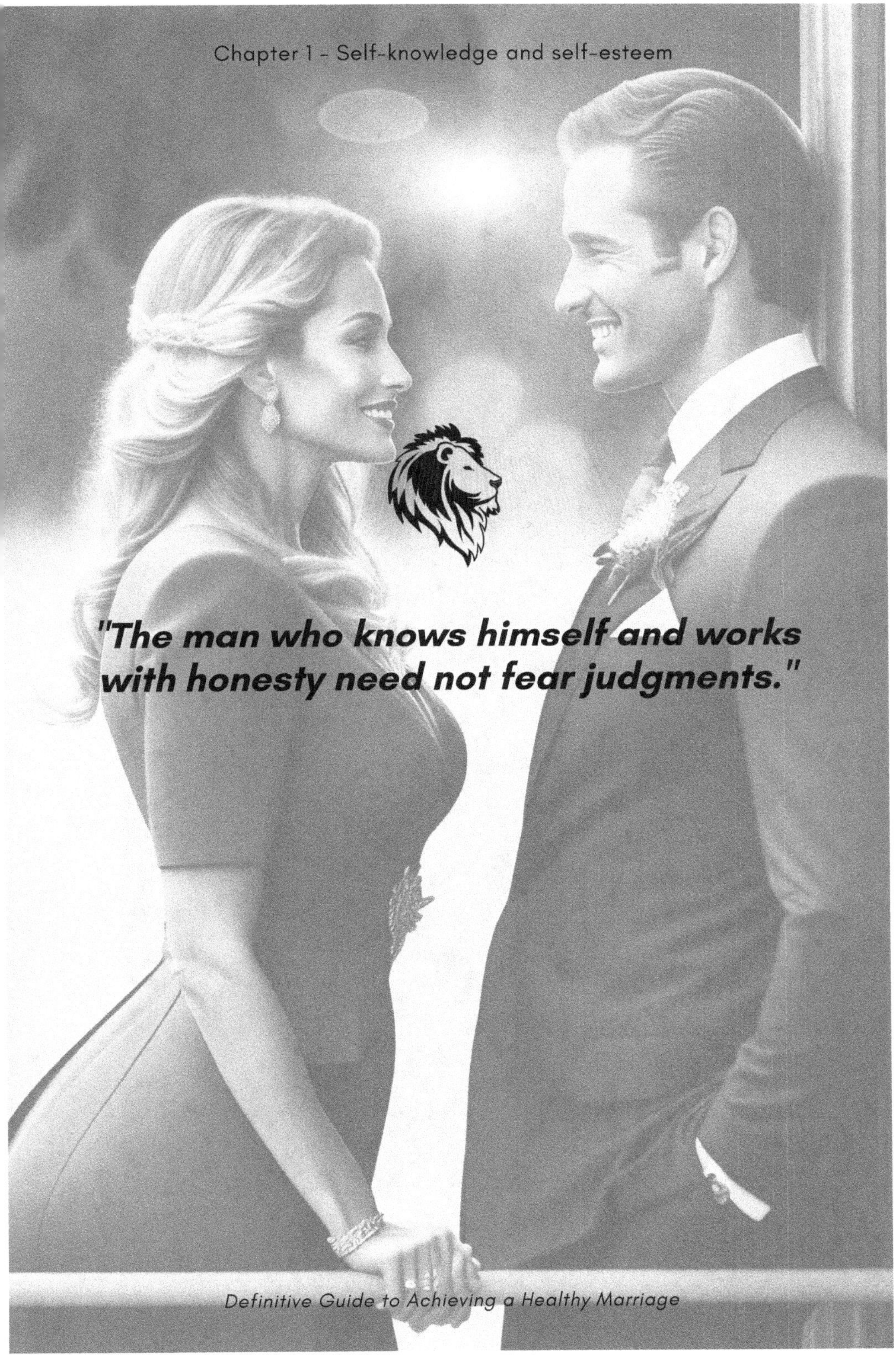

"The man who knows himself and works with honesty need not fear judgments."

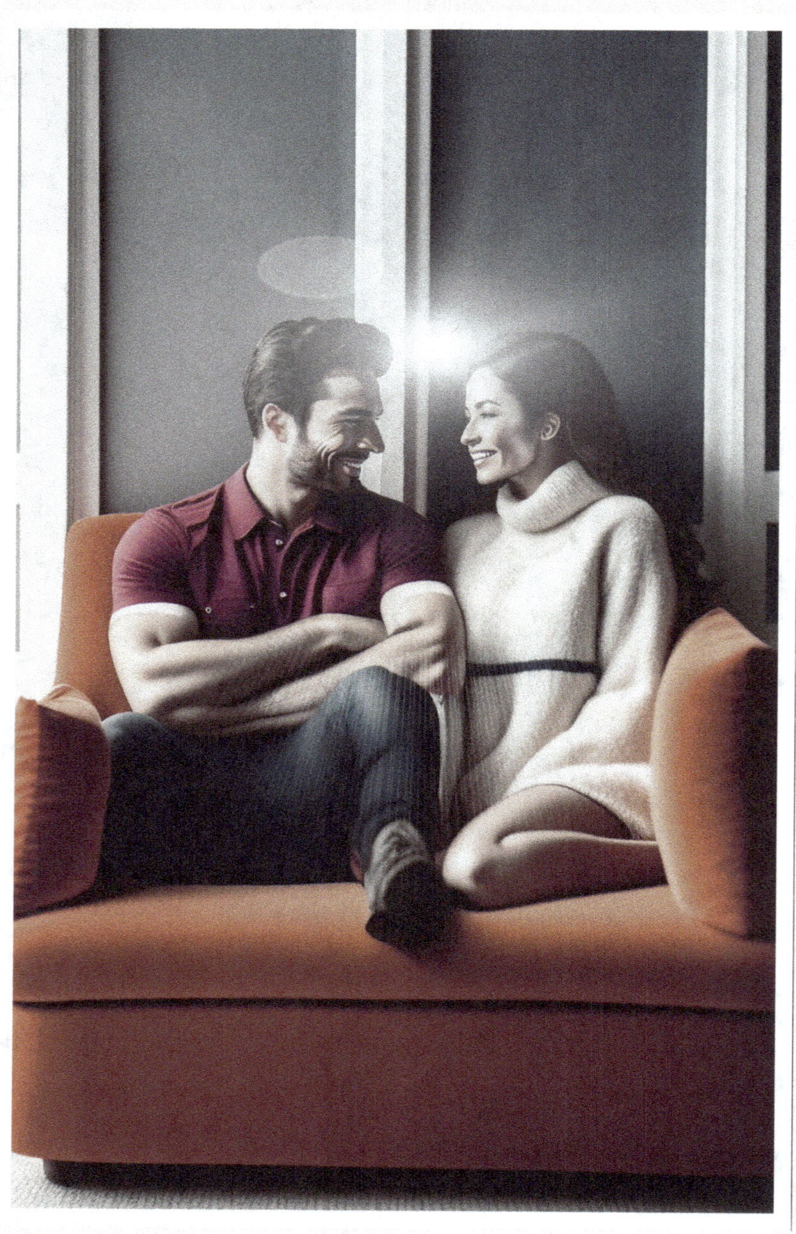

Effective communication

The importance of effective communication in marriage

Communication is essential for any relationship, and marriage is no different. Effective communication is critical to success and happiness in marriage.

When partners communicate openly, clearly, and respectfully, they can build a stronger, healthier relationship. Communication is also important for resolving conflicts, making decisions, and sharing feelings and thoughts.

On the other hand, inadequate communication can lead to misunderstandings, resentments, frustrations, and conflicts. It's important to remember that effective communication is not just talking, but also actively listening and understanding your partner's needs and feelings.

In this chapter, we'll discuss the importance of communication and provide tips and exercises to help you develop your communication skills.

Tips and exercises to improve communication with your partner:

- **Practice active listening:** pay attention to what your partner is saying and try to understand their feelings and needs. Ask questions and repeat what you heard to ensure you understood correctly.

- **Be surgical:** use clear and objective language to avoid misunderstandings. Avoid using words that can be interpreted in different ways.

- **Don't interrupt your partner:** Allow your partner to express their thoughts and feelings without interruption. Wait until she has finished talking before responding.

- **Use "I" instead of "you":** When expressing your needs and feelings, use sentences that start with "I" instead of "you". For example, instead of saying "You never listen to me", say "I feel like I'm not being heard".

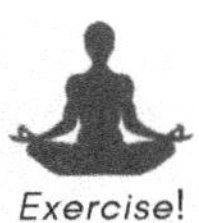

Exercise!

- **Practice conflict resolution:** When there is a conflict, try to resolve it constructively. Avoid blaming your partner and try to find a solution that works for both of you.

- **Make time to talk:** Make time to talk every day, even if it's just for a few minutes. It will help you connect and share your thoughts and feelings.

By practicing these tips and exercises, you will be improving communication in your marriage and building stronger, healthier relationships.

Remember that communication is a skill that can be learned and improved with practice.

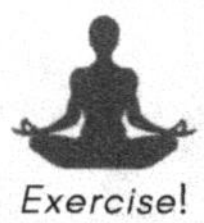

Exercise!

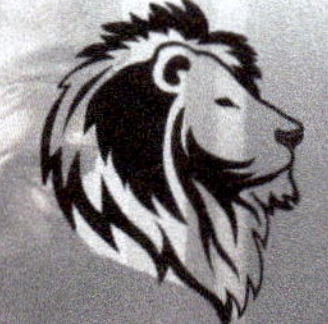

"Communicating feelings is for the strong. The weak don't have that courage."

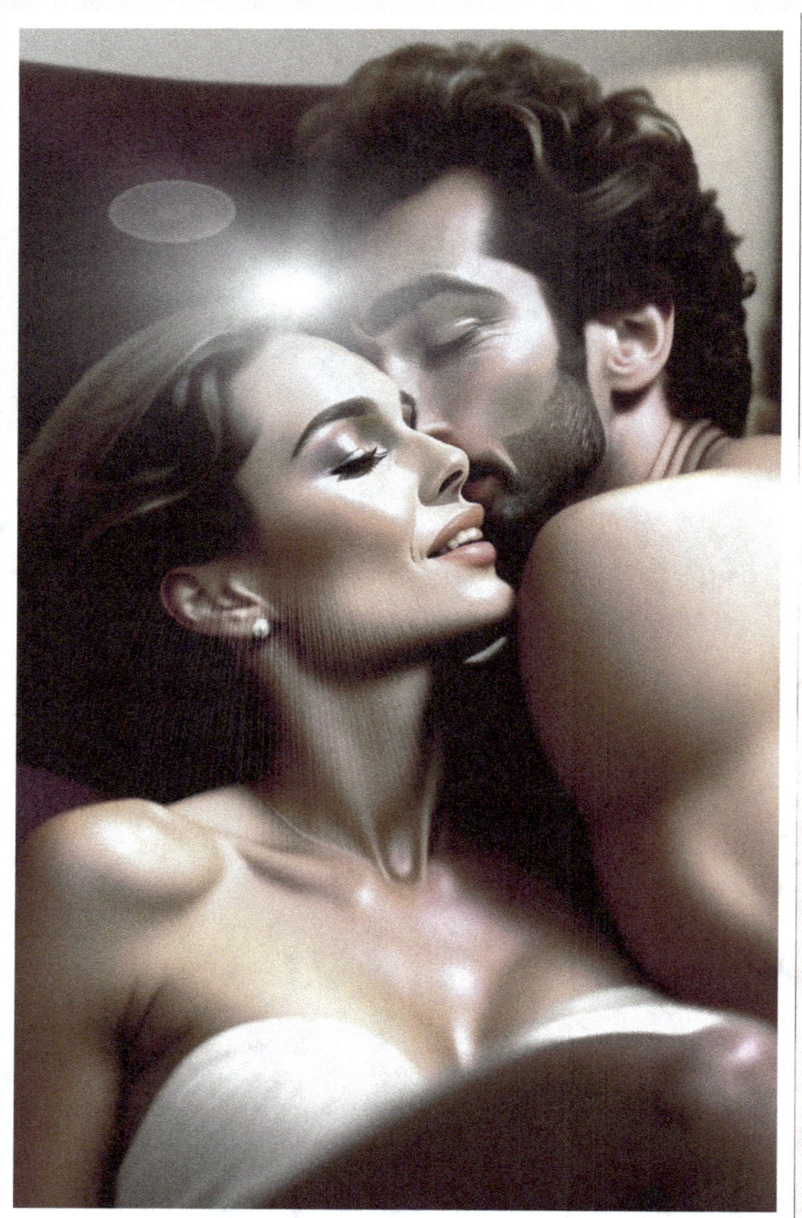

Empathy

What is empathy and how can it help build a healthy marriage

Empathy is the ability to put yourself in another's shoes and understand their feelings and perspectives. In the context of marriage, empathy can help build a healthier and more loving relationship, as it allows partners to understand and support each other.

When you are empathetic to your partner, you can understand how they feel in a given situation and thus respond accordingly. This can help you avoid conflict and build a stronger connection between you.

Tips and exercises to develop empathy:

- **Practice active listening:** when your partner talks, pay attention to what he is saying. Try to understand her feelings and perspective.

- **Put yourself in the other person's shoes:** imagine how you would feel if you were in your partner's situation. This can help her better understand your feelings and perspectives.

- **Be patient:** It's not always easy to understand each other's emotions and perspectives. Be patient and keep trying.

- **Consider individual differences:** Remember that each person has their own story and life experiences. Try to understand how these differences can affect your partner's emotions and outlook.

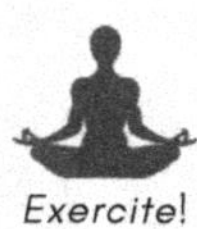

Exercite!

- **Practice gratitude:** Acknowledge the good things your partner does for you and show gratitude. This can help build a more loving and empathetic relationship.

By developing empathy in your relationship, you will be building a strong foundation for a healthy and loving marriage. Remember that empathy is a skill that can be developed and improved with time and practice.

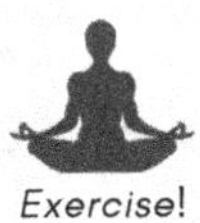

Exercise!

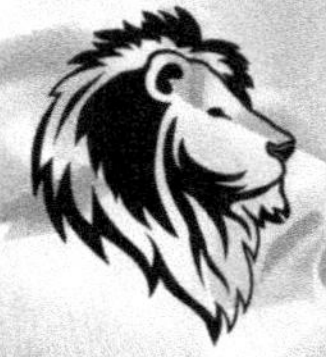

"Immersing yourself in the universe of others is essential to make an important part of your life."

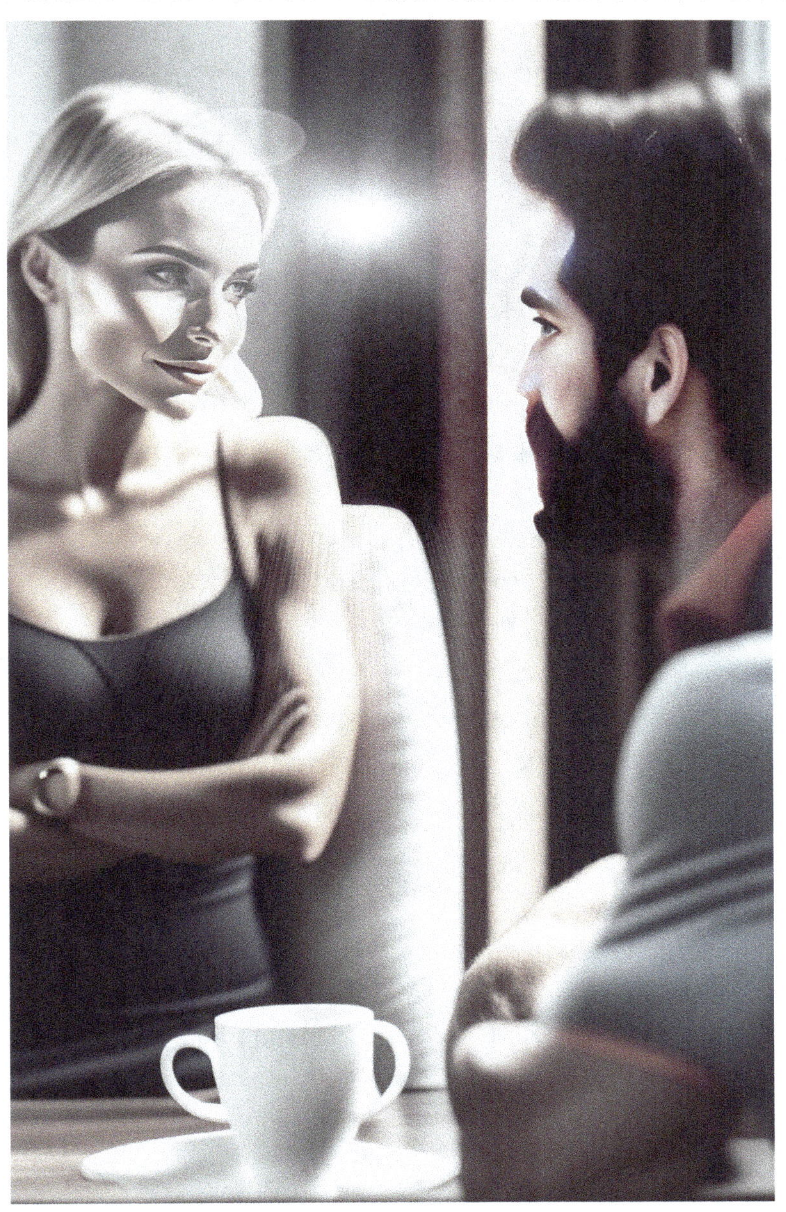

How Emotional Intelligence Can Help Build a Healthy Marriage

Emotional intelligence is the ability to understand and manage our own emotions, as well as understand and respond to the emotions of others. In the context of marriage, emotional intelligence can help build a healthy and loving relationship.

It can help improve mutual understanding between you and your partner, allowing you to better understand each other's emotions and perspectives.

Developing emotional intelligence can help communication between you and your partner, allowing you to express your feelings clearly and objectively.

Conflicts are resolved in a very constructive and healthy way by developing this skill. This makes it more feasible to work together to find mutually satisfactory solutions.

Tips and exercises to develop emotional intelligence:

- **Practice self-awareness:** Try to understand and identify your own emotions. This can help you manage them more effectively and understand how they affect your behavior and decisions.

- **Practice empathy:** Try to understand your partner's emotions and perspectives. This can help you respond more appropriately and effectively to her emotional needs.

- **Develop Emotion Regulation:** Try to find healthy ways to manage your own emotions. This can include activities such as exercise, meditation, or therapy.

- **Practice Effective Communication:** Work on the ability to communicate clearly and objectively. This may involve using phrases that begin with "I" instead of "you", which can help to avoid guilt and hostility.

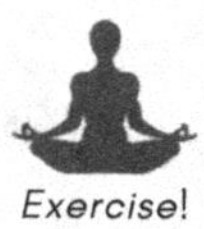

Exercise!

- **Be open to feedback:** Be willing to receive constructive feedback from your partner and work on areas where you can improve your emotional intelligence.

By developing emotional intelligence in your relationship, you will be building a solid foundation for a healthy and loving marriage. Remember that emotional intelligence is a skill that can be developed and improved with time and practice.

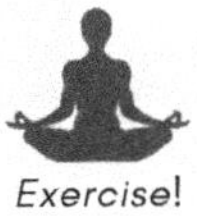

Exercise!

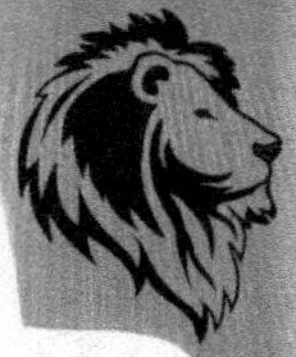

"*Emotions come from internal triggers. Understanding and transcending these triggers is maturing. The mature man owns his emotions.*"

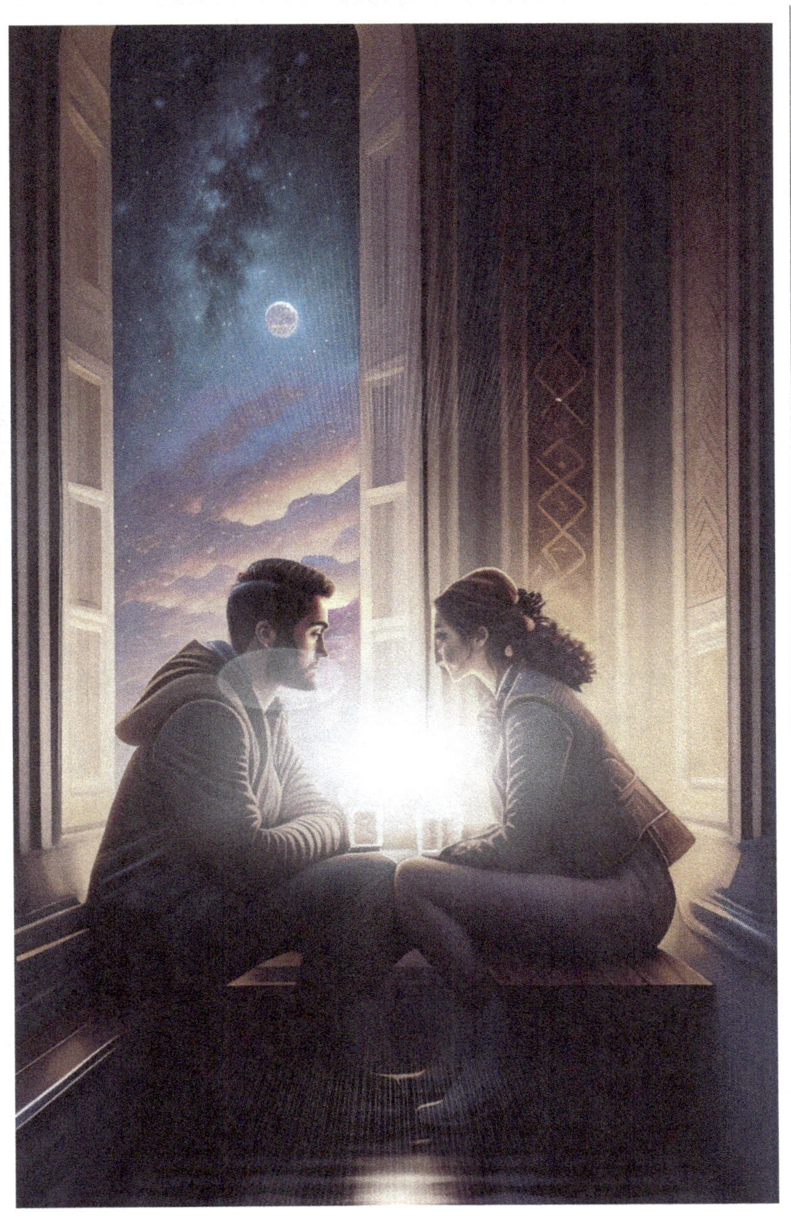

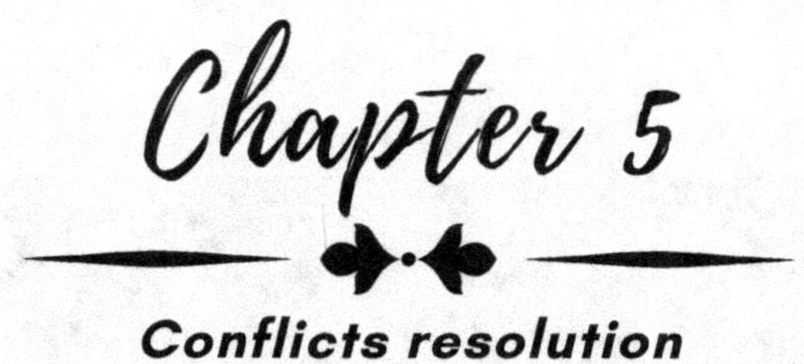

Conflicts resolution

The importance of conflict resolution in marriage

Conflicts are inevitable in any relationship. When you know how to resolve conflicts effectively, you can strengthen your relationship and increase your intimacy with your partner.

Conflict resolution can help build trust, understanding, and connection between you and your partner.

In this chapter, we'll discuss the importance of conflict resolution and provide tips and exercises to help you develop this skill.

Tips and exercises to resolve conflicts in a constructive and healthy way:

- **Talk about your feelings:** Try to express your feelings clearly and objectively. Avoid blaming your partner and use phrases that start with "I". For example, instead of saying "You're always wrong", say "I get frustrated when we can't come to an agreement".

- **Listen Empathetically:** Try to understand your partner's feelings and perspectives. Pay attention to what he is saying and try to see things from her point of view.

- **Find a mutually satisfactory solution:** Work with your partner to find a mutually satisfactory solution. Be creative and be willing to compromise.

- **Don't avoid conflict:** Avoid avoiding conflict and pretending everything is fine. This can lead to resentment and an unhealthy relationship.

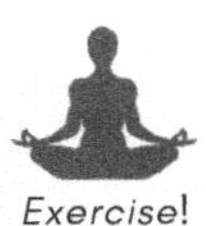

Exercise!

- **Apologize when necessary:** If you're wrong, apologize. This can help rebuild trust and connection in your relationship.

By resolving conflicts constructively and healthily, you will be strengthening your relationship and building a solid foundation for a happy and healthy marriage.

Remember that conflict resolution is a skill that can be honed and developed with time and practice.

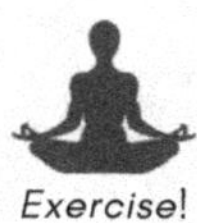

Exercise!

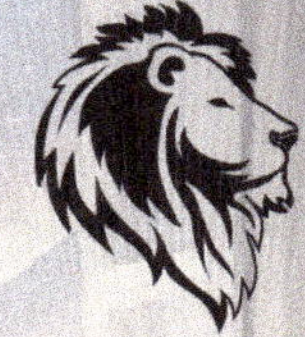

"Unlike many aspects of peace, conflict is a great opportunity for a couple to grow."

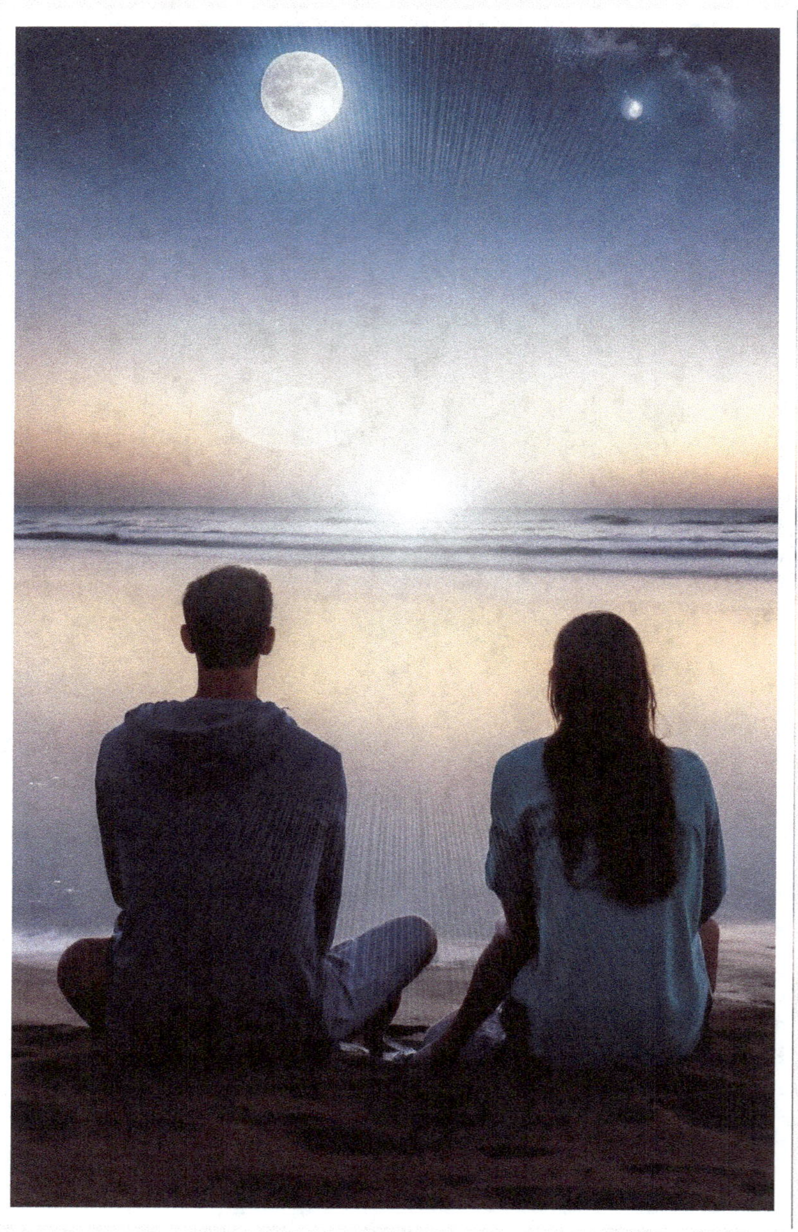

Chapter 6

Dealing with anger

How to Deal with Anger and Have a Healthy Marriage

Knowing how to deal with anger is essential to maintain healthy relationships and avoid unnecessary conflicts. Anger is a normal and natural emotion, but when not properly controlled it can lead to destructive behaviors such as physical or verbal aggression, isolation, resentment, and hostility. In addition, anger can negatively affect physical and emotional health, causing stress, anxiety, and related illnesses such as high blood pressure and heart disease.

By learning to deal with anger in healthy ways, you can improve communication with your partner, resolve conflicts more effectively, and develop stronger, more loving relationships.

In addition, you will learn to better manage your own emotions, improving your physical and emotional health and becoming a happier and more fulfilled person.

In short, dealing with anger healthily is an essential skill for a happy, healthy relationship and a full, satisfying life.

Tips and exercises for dealing with anger healthily in your relationship with your wife:

- **Listen carefully:** Many times, anger can arise due to misunderstandings and miscommunication. Try to listen carefully to what your wife is saying and ask questions to clarify any doubts. This can help to avoid misunderstandings that can lead to anger.

- **Be honest:** If you feel angry, try to express your feelings honestly and objectively. Communicate your needs and expectations clearly, but without blaming your wife. Remember to use sentences that start with "I" instead of "you".

- **Take a deep breath:** When you feel anger rising, try taking a few deep breaths before responding. This can help you calm down and avoid saying or doing something impulsive.

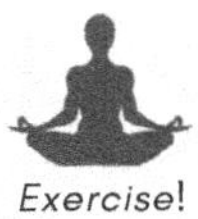

Exercise!

- **Practice empathy:** Try to understand your wife's emotions and perspective. This can help you respond more appropriately and effectively to her emotional needs.

- **Find activities to release tension:** Find activities that help release tension, such as exercise, meditation, or writing in a journal.

- **Consider therapy:** If you feel that anger is hurting your relationship, consider seeking professional help. A therapist can help you develop skills to deal with anger healthily.

By dealing with anger in healthy ways in your relationship with your wife, you will be strengthening your marriage and building a strong foundation for a happy and healthy future together.

Remember that anger is a normal emotion, but it's important to manage it in a healthy way to avoid emotional and physical harm.

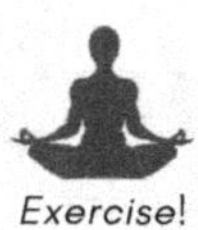

Exercise!

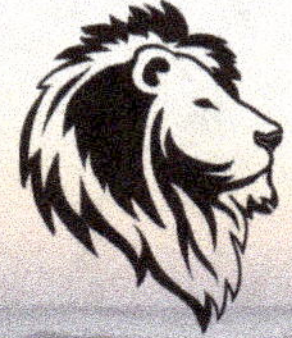

"The well-channeled anger is one of the greatest strengths we can have."

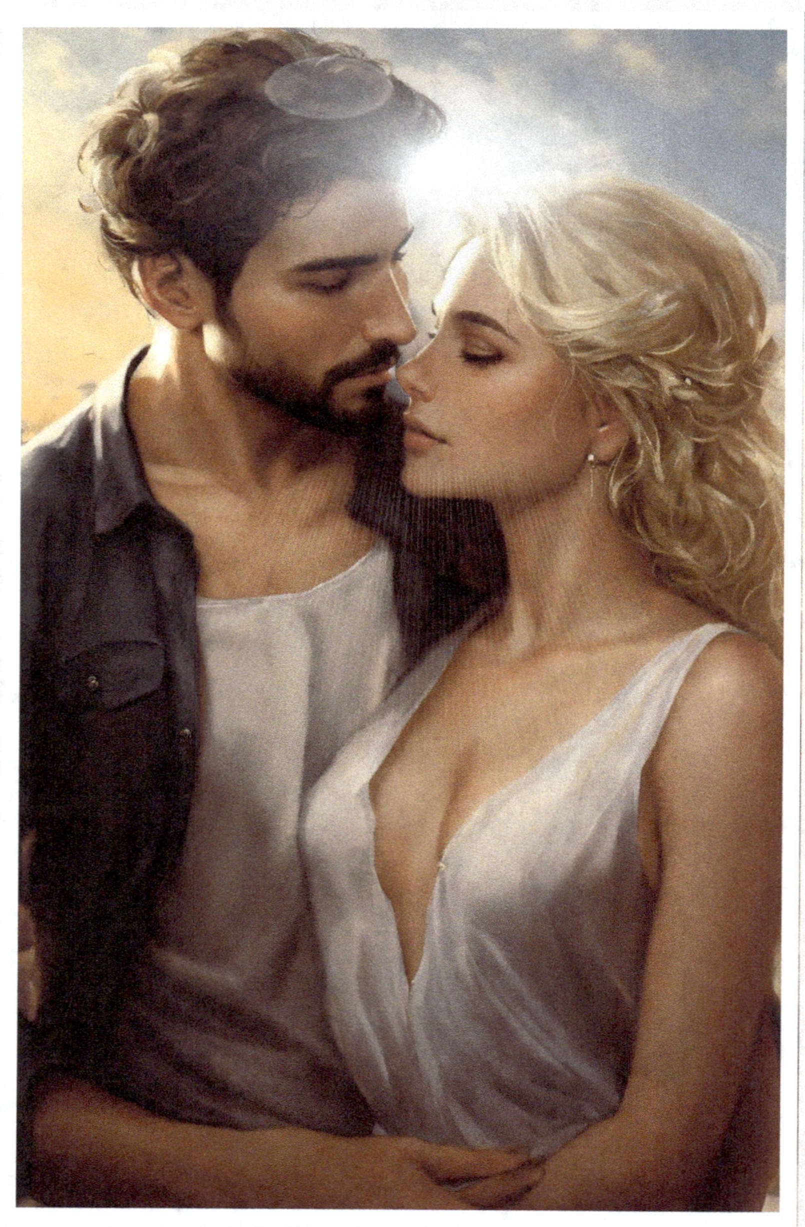

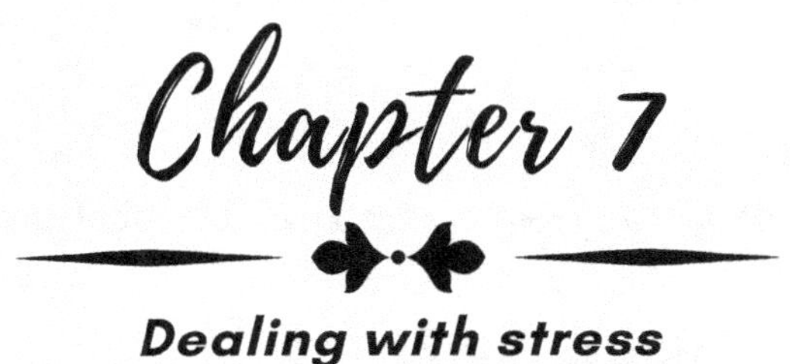

Chapter 7

Dealing with stress

How to Deal with Marriage Stress

Stress is an inevitable part of life and can affect any relationship. When stress is not managed properly, it can lead to conflict, resentment, and health problems.

However, there are many ways to deal with stress healthily in a relationship.

In this chapter, we'll discuss some tips and exercises to help you deal with stress in your relationship.

Tips and exercises to deal with stress:

- **Communicate Clearly:** It is important that you and your partner communicate clearly about what is causing stress in your lives. When you can share your worries and anxieties with your partner, it can help ease the burden of stress. Also, it can help them work together to find solutions to their problems.

- **Practice empathy: You and your partner need to empathize** with each other during times of stress. When you put yourself in your partner's shoes, it can help reduce tension and anxiety. Remember that stress affects people in different ways, and being empathetic can help you emotionally connect and support each other.

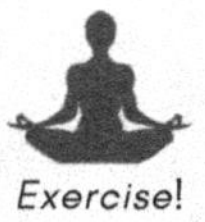

Exercise!

- **Take regular breaks:** When you're under stress, it's important to take regular breaks to take care of yourself. This could include a break from work, a walk, or just sitting and relaxing for a few minutes. Remember that taking care of yourself is an important part of managing stress.

Dealing with stress in a relationship can be challenging, but it is possible. Clear communication, practicing empathy, finding activities that help reduce stress, taking regular breaks, and considering therapy are all effective ways to deal with stress in your relationship.

Remember that stress is a normal part of life, but it's important to manage it in a healthy way to maintain a happy and healthy relationship.

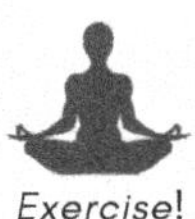

Exercise!

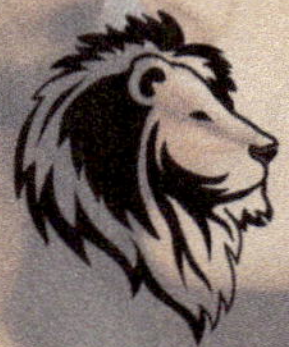

"Fear is the predecessor of stress. Fear in balance is healthy. Stress is fear waiting to be overcome."

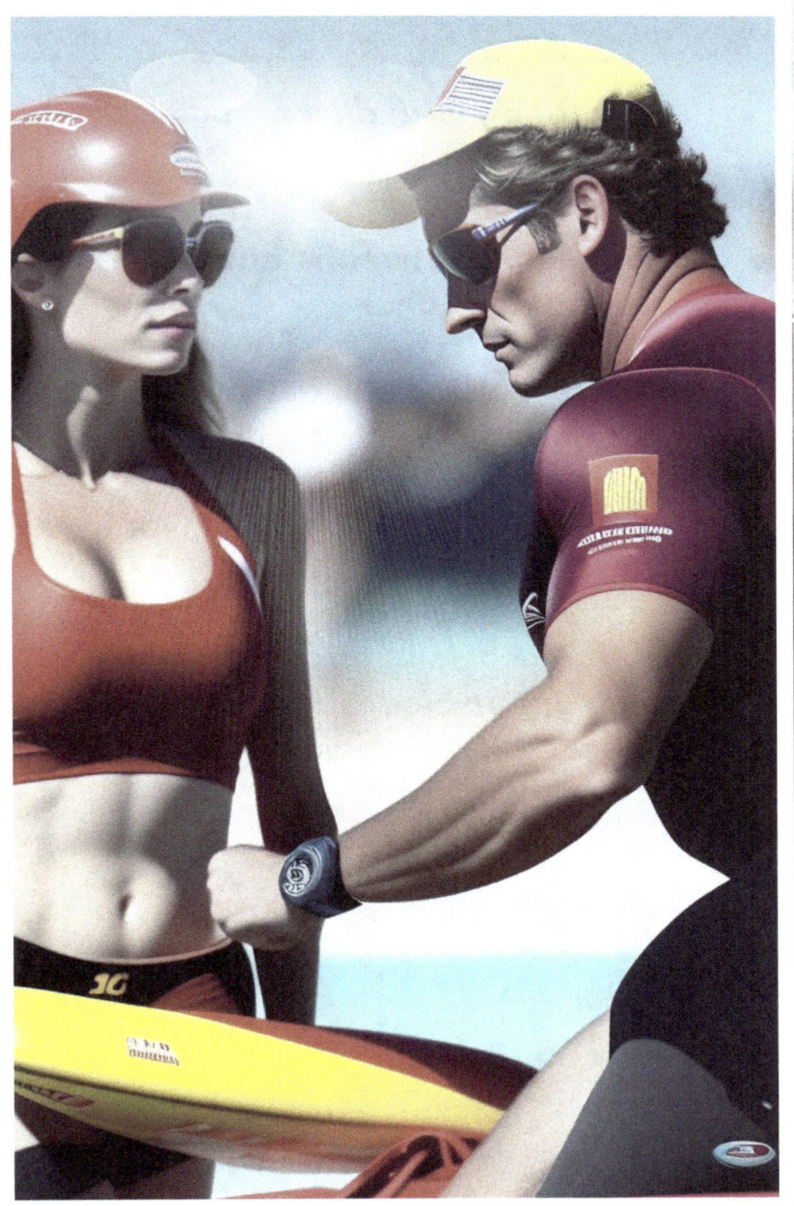

Dealing with differences

The relationship between differences and conflicts in the relationship

Differences are inevitable in any relationship, but they are not always easy to deal with. When they are not properly resolved, they can generate conflicts and tensions in the relationship.

In this chapter, we will discuss the relationship between differences and conflict in relationships and give tips and exercises for dealing with this great skill needed in all areas of life, especially in marriage.

Tips and exercises for dealing with differences:

- **Respectful Freedom:** It's important that you and your partner can express your opinions and feelings openly and respectfully. Try to understand your partner's point of view and be willing to compromise.

- **Find common ground:** While you may have different opinions about certain things, it is possible to find common ground. Try to find activities that you both enjoy doing together and that you can enjoy together.

Finally, it's important to remember that differences don't have to be a sign of problems in the relationship. They can be an opportunity to learn more about your partner and grow together.

By handling differences healthily, you can strengthen your relationship and build a solid foundation for a happy and healthy future together.

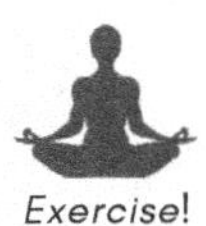

Exercise!

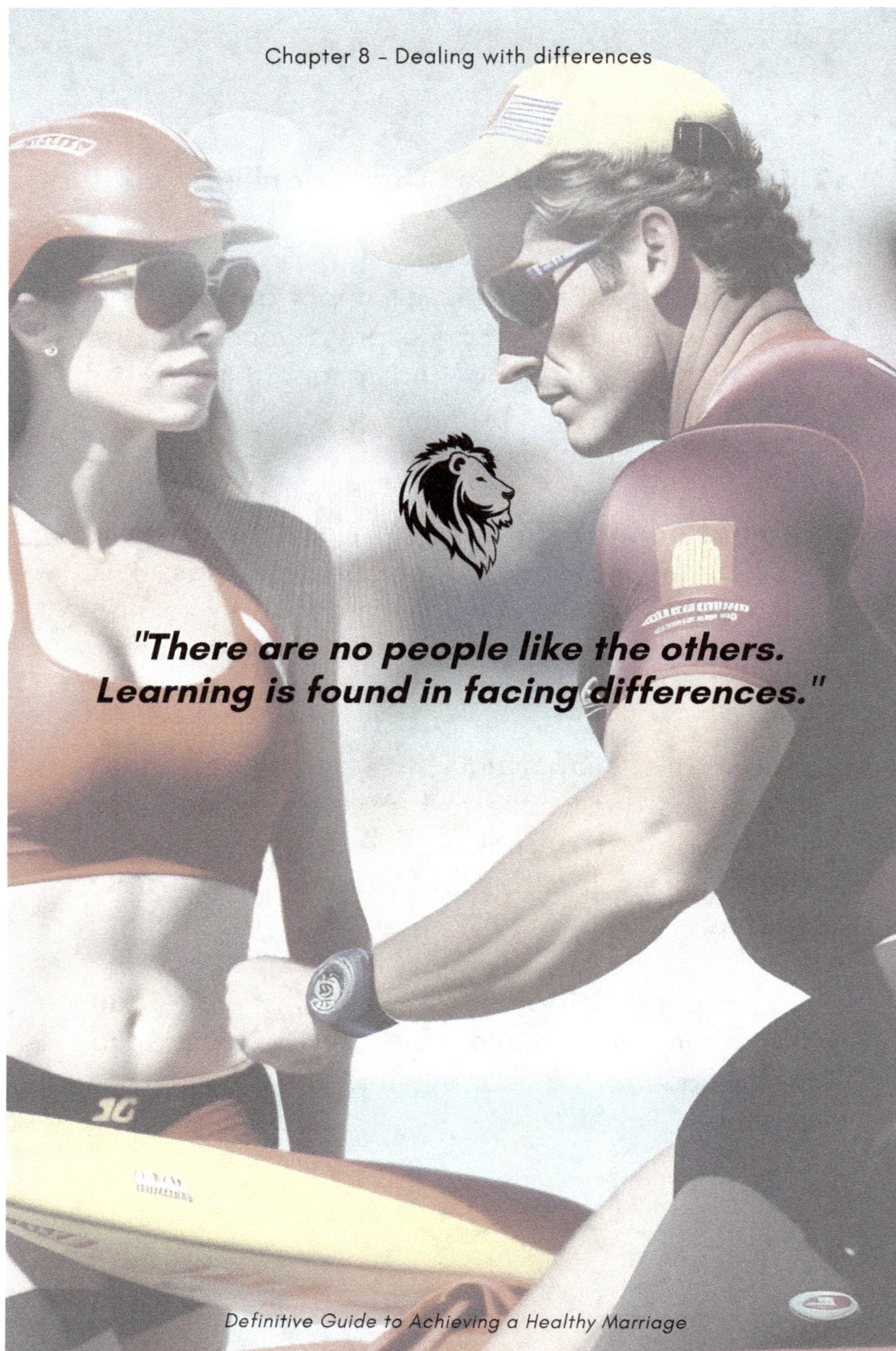

Chapter 8 – Dealing with differences
"There are no people like the others.
Learning is found in facing differences."
Definitive Guide to Achieving a Healthy Marriage

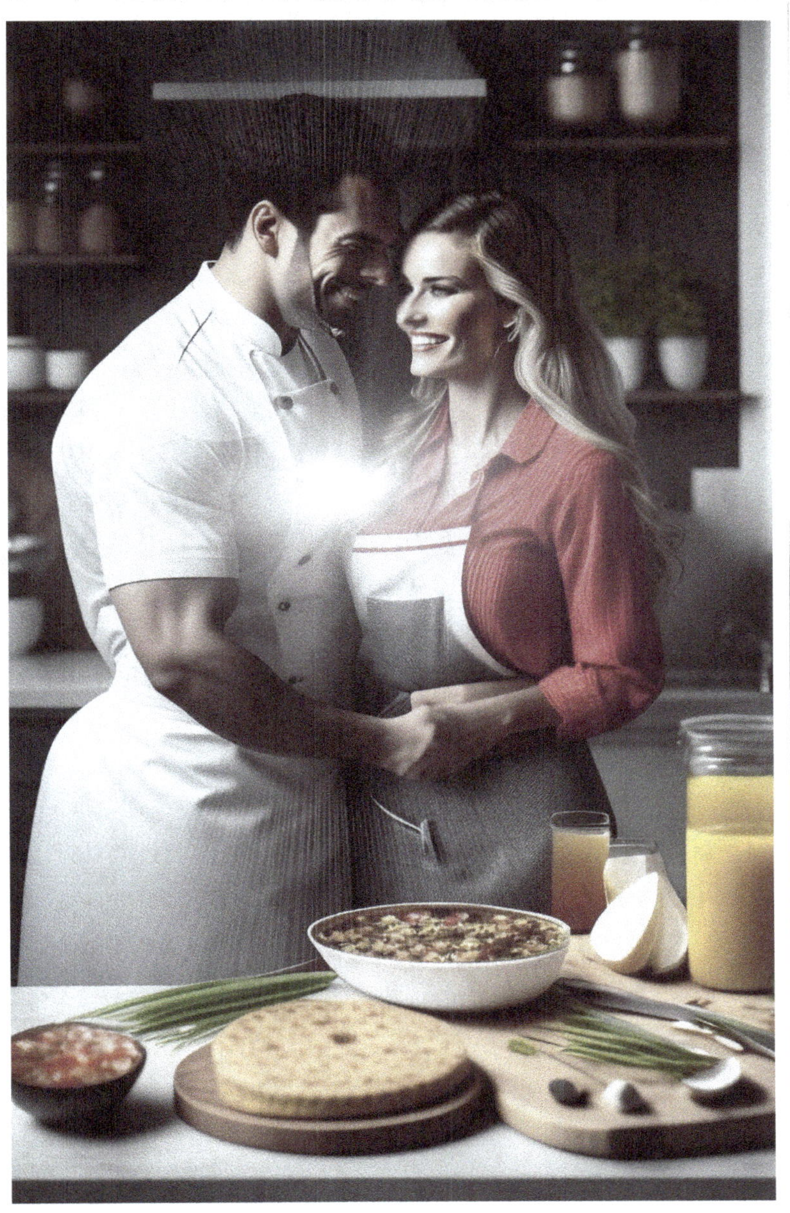

Dealing with expectations

The relationship between expectations and disappointments in the relationship

Expectations are a natural part of any relationship. We all have expectations of our partner and the relationship itself. However, when these expectations are not met, it can lead to disappointment and conflict.

It is noteworthy that expectations are one of the greatest sources of anxiety and suffering. Therefore, pay close attention to this topic.

In this chapter, we'll discuss the relationship between expectations and disappointments in a relationship and provide tips and exercises for dealing with this dilemma.

Tips and exercises for dealing with expectations:

- **Understand your desires:** First, try to understand what you expect from the relationship and the rest of your life. Dive deep within yourself and find your truth. This is the only way to share clear and complete information.

- **Negotiate:** Try to understand your partner's point of view and be willing to compromise. Always seek a more advanced balance for you and your marriage. This is very relevant in relationships and produces very good complicity.

- **Be realistic about your expectations:** It's important to remember that no relationship is perfect and that both partners have flaws and imperfections. Try to be flexible and willing to adjust your expectations as the relationship evolves.

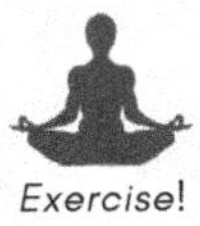

Exercise!

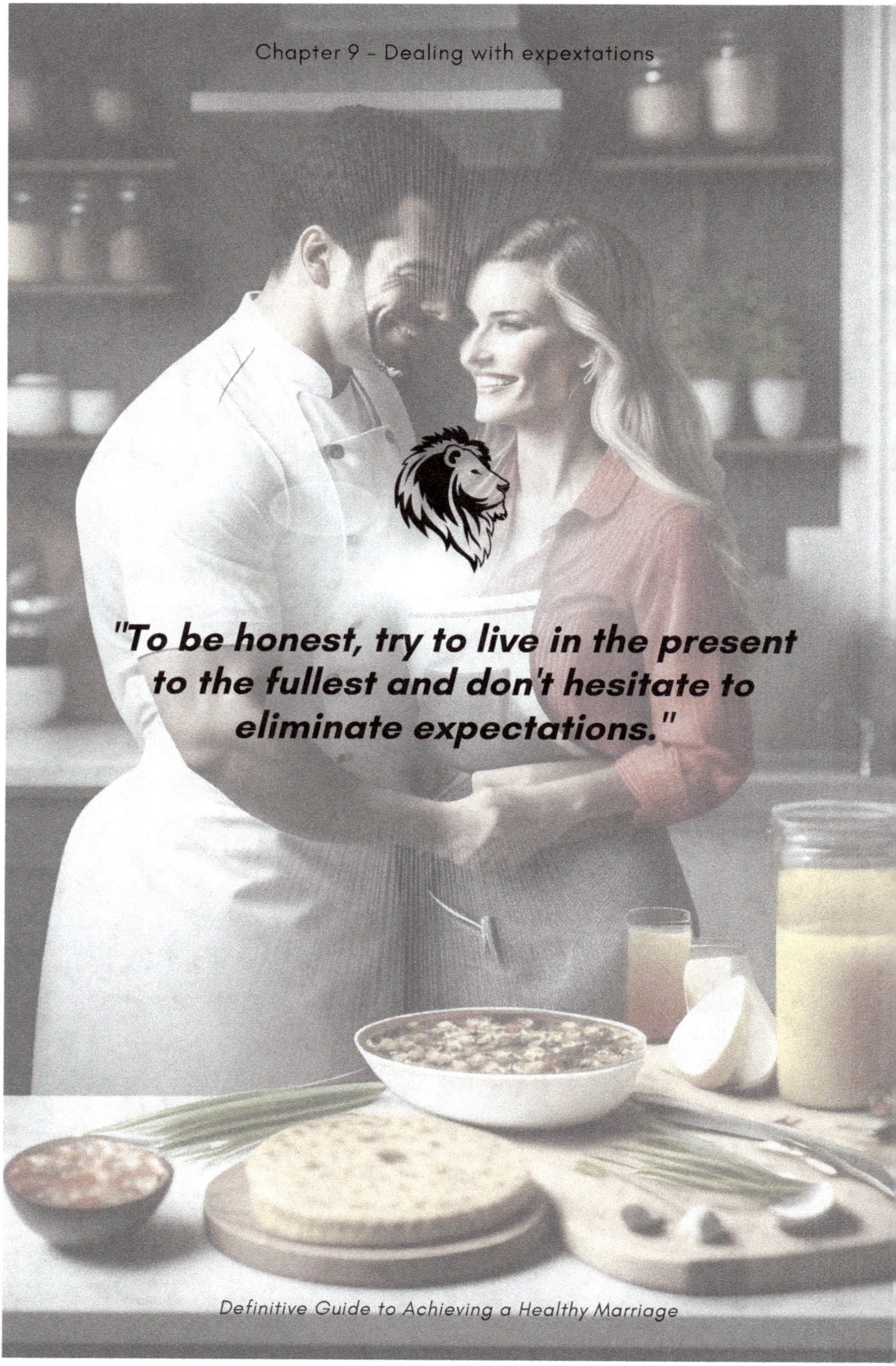

"*To be honest, try to live in the present to the fullest and don't hesitate to eliminate expectations.*"

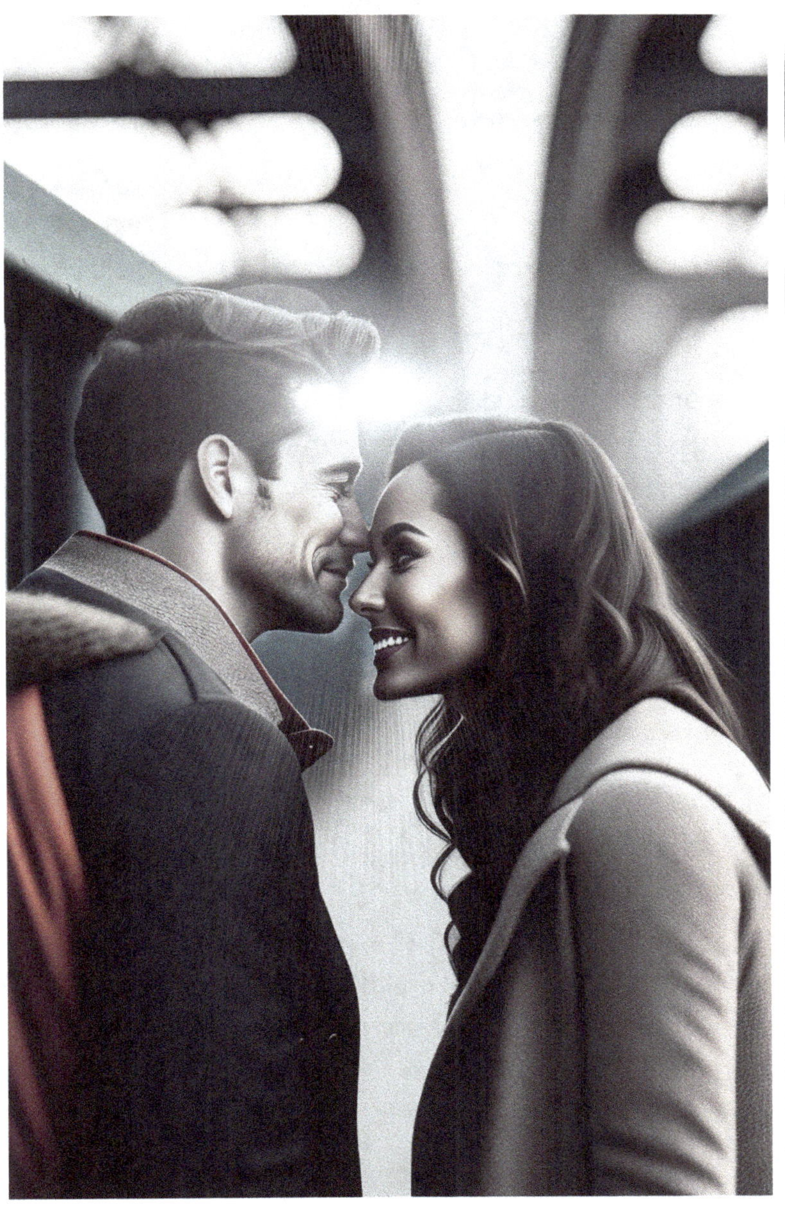

The importance of forgiveness

Definition of forgiveness and its importance to the relationship

Forgiveness is an important part of any relationship. When failures and mistakes happen, it's important to be able to forgive and move on. This is a virtue, which can be considered one of the most important, capable of releasing anger and resentment against someone who has hurt us.

Forgiveness doesn't mean you're accepting the behavior or minimizing the harm done. Rather, forgiveness is a conscious choice to let go of the past and move forward.

In this chapter, we will discuss the definition of forgiveness and its importance to marriage. In addition, we will give tips and exercises to develop forgiveness.

Tips and exercises to learn to forgive:

- **Practice empathy:** When you can understand your partner's point of view and the reasons behind their behaviors, forgiving will become easier and more natural. Because when there are no resentments and anger, the connection becomes much healthier.

- **Assume your part in the situation:** Express your feelings clearly and truthfully. Understand that you have been hurt and that you have negative feelings, and convey your understanding. This is a key factor in being able to focus on how you feel instead of blaming your partner.

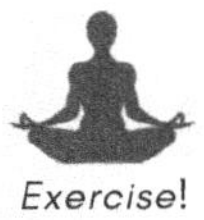

Exercise!

Finally, it is important to remember that forgiveness is a process. It can take time and effort to get to a place of forgiveness. If you are struggling to forgive, it may be helpful to seek professional help. A therapist can help you develop strategies for dealing with anger and resentment and help you find a way to move forward.

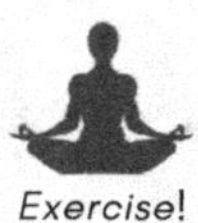

Exercise!

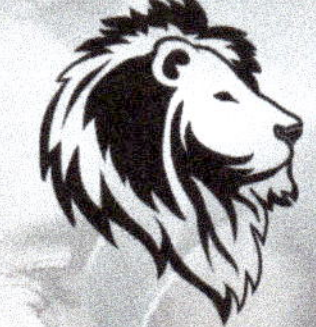

"Forgiving is smart and opens the flow for progress. Now remember that forgetting is stupid and makes you miss out on learning."

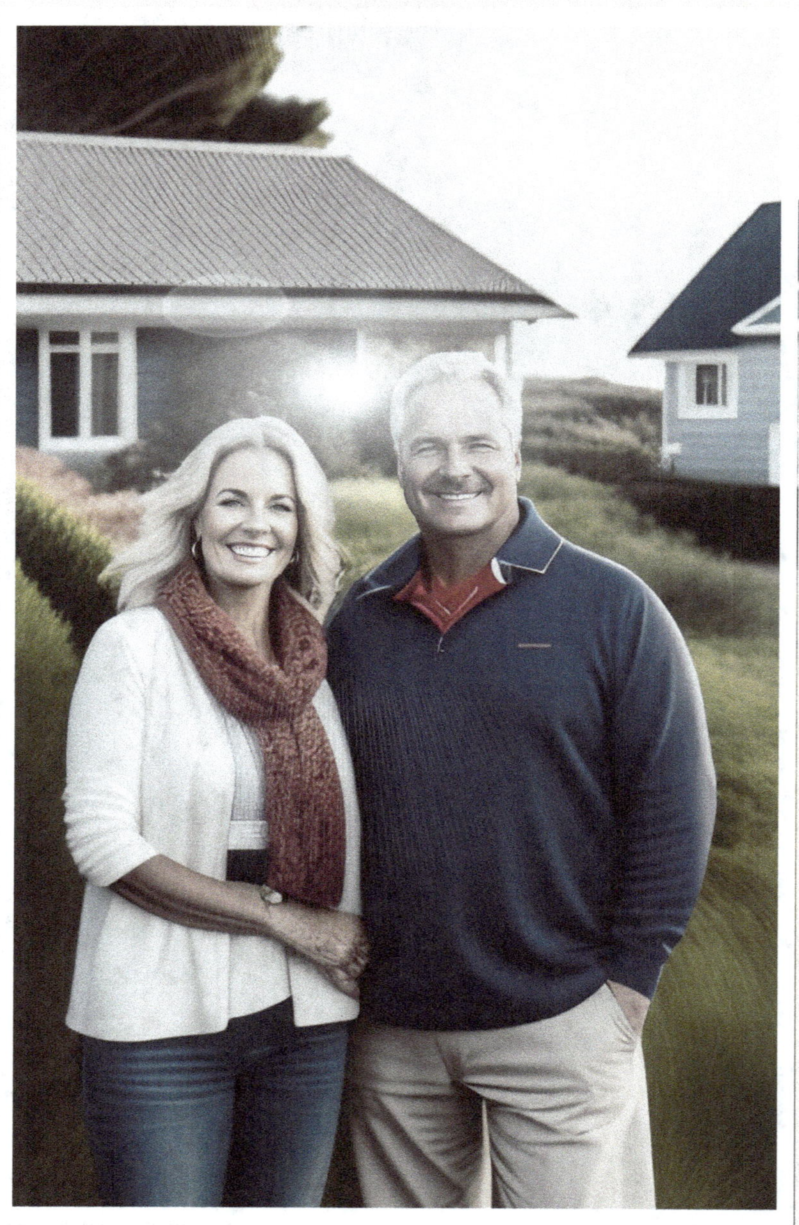

Chapter 11

Dealing with the routine

The relationship between routine and monotony in the relationship

Routine is an inevitable part of any relationship. Over time, things can become monotonous and predictable. However, the routine can also be a challenge for the relationship. In this chapter, we'll discuss the relationship between routine and monotony in a relationship and provide tips and exercises for dealing with routine.

Some routines do well, as they are fundamental, such as taking care of the children, organizing finances, and having dinner together. However, there are also unhealthy routines that create apathy in marriage. The name of this is "comfort zone". Filtering this out is important for the desired health of the marriage.

Here are some tips on how to deal with the routine:

- **Simple attitudes:** One of the first things you can do to deal with routine is to focus on the little things. Try to find ways to surprise your partner and keep things interesting. This could include romantic surprises, a warm conversation, matters that require concentration and judgment from both of you or simply doing something out of the ordinary.

- **Open communication:** Another important tip is to keep communication open. When things become routine, it can be easy to stop communicating. However, it's important that you and your partner can openly talk about your feelings and needs.

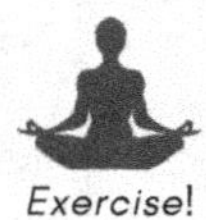

Exercise!

Finally, it's important to remember that change is a natural part of life. Sometimes routine can be a sign that it's time to make changes in your life and your relationship. Be open to new experiences and try to find ways to grow and evolve together.

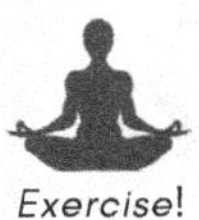

Exercise!

"*Routine is essential for stability in a marriage.*"

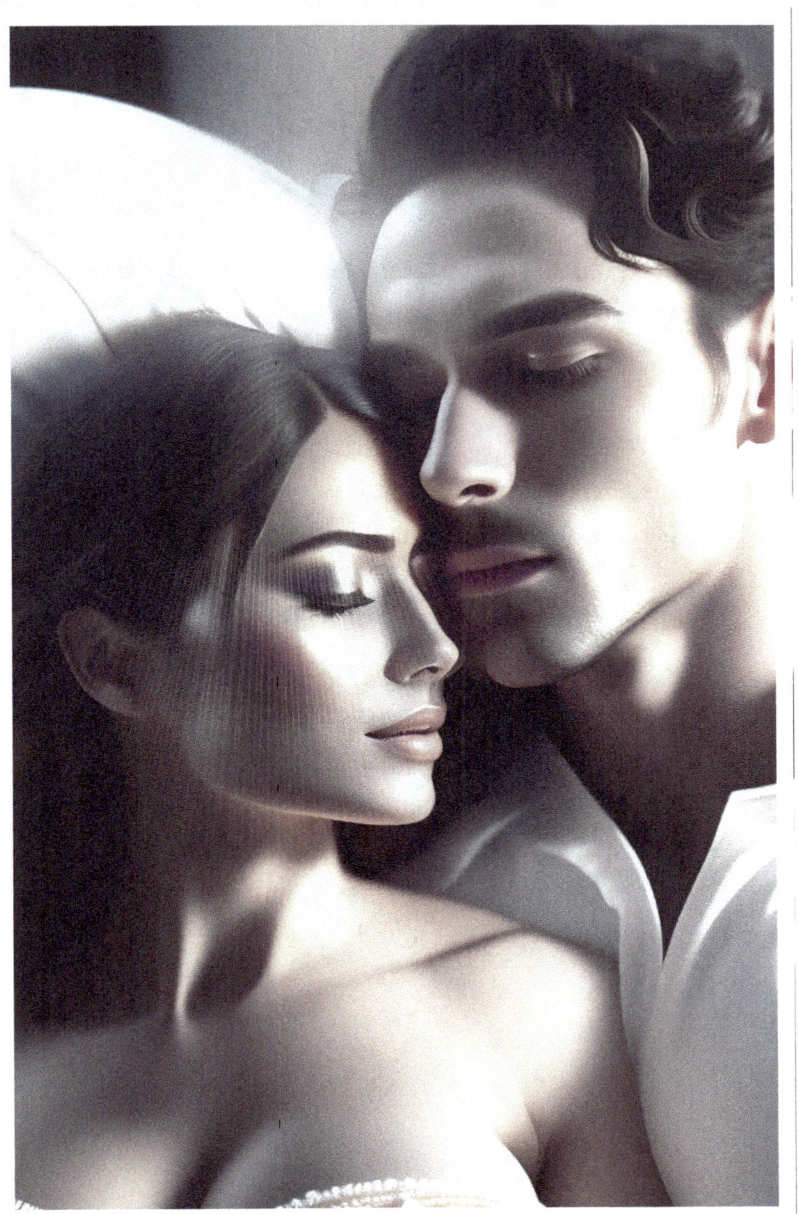

Chapter 12

Keeping the passion

The relationship between passion and intimacy in the relationship

Passion is an important part of any relationship. However, maintaining passion can be a challenge over time. In this chapter, we'll discuss the relationship between passion and intimacy in a relationship and provide tips and exercises for maintaining passion.

Passion in marriage is simply living with the enthusiasm of growing together, of feeling loved and cherished. A marriage with stimuli for professional, personal, spiritual, and sexual growth grows and prospers because, through healthy passion, everyday life becomes light and productive.

Here are some tips for living with healthy passion in marriage:

- **Emotional Intimacy:** One of the first things you can do to maintain passion is to focus on emotional intimacy. As time passes, it can be easy to lose your emotional connection with your partner. Try to find ways to connect emotionally with deep conversations, allowing yourself vulnerability and sharing your feelings.

- **Romantic Surprises:** Create moments like romantic surprises, taking trips together, or trying new things in bed.

Finally, it's important to remember that passion can be cultivated. You can learn to be more passionate and find ways to keep the passion alive in your relationship. Be open to new experiences and try to find ways to grow and evolve together.

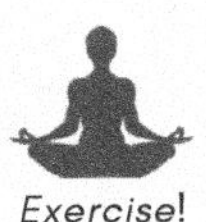

Exercise!

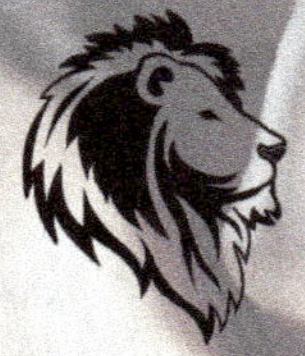

"*Your passion should always be for ideas that thrive.*"

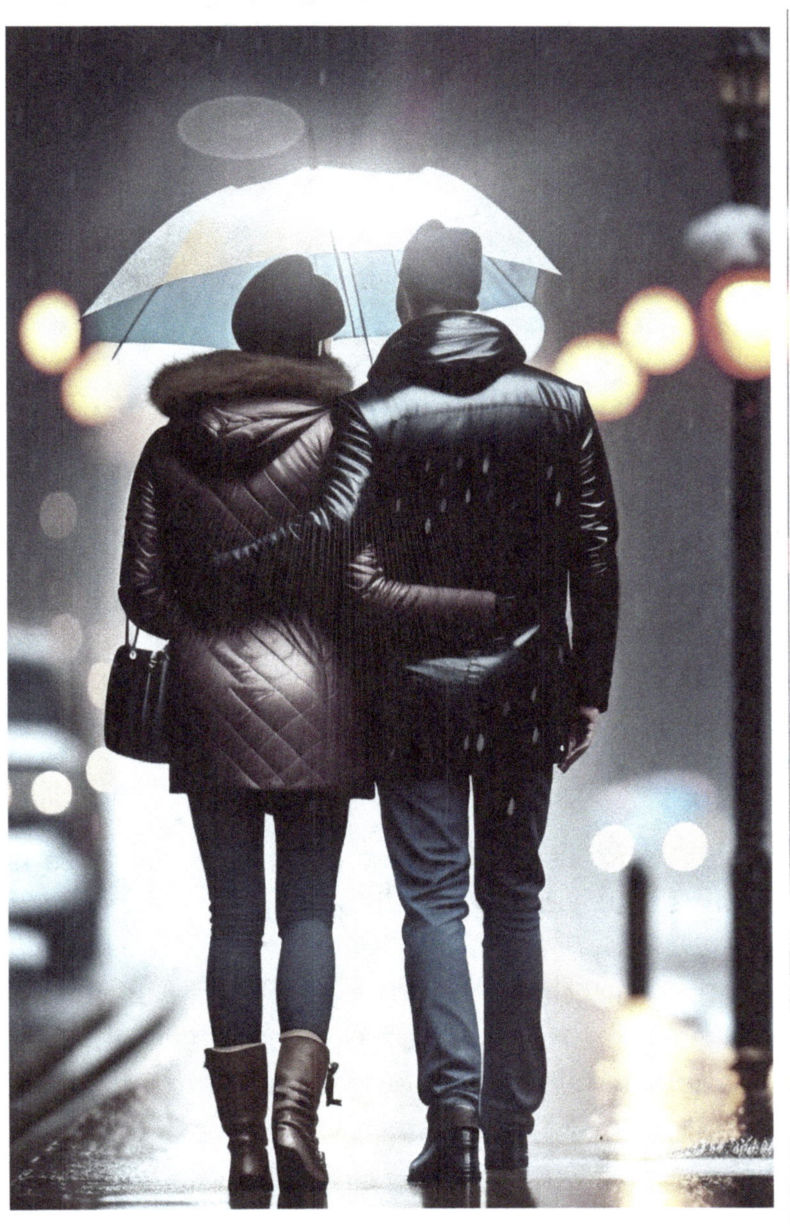

Chapter 13

Cultivating gratitude

Definition of gratitude and its importance to the relationship

Gratitude is an important part of any relationship. When we are grateful, we are better able to appreciate the good things in our lives and our relationships. In this chapter, we'll discuss the definition of gratitude and its importance to a relationship. In addition, we will give tips and exercises to cultivate gratitude. This can help strengthen the emotional connection between the two of you.

We must understand that practicing gratitude is a fundamental part of well-being. In everything in life, to know how to value, we need to be grateful. This does not mean that we should like everything that happens to us, but that we should know how to filter the best of each situation.

Here are some tips on how to experience gratitude for a healthy marriage:

- **Gratitude Journal:** One of the first things you can do to cultivate gratitude is to keep a gratitude journal. Try writing down a few things you are grateful for every day. This could include things like your partner's characteristics, your health, your family, or your job.

- **Express Yourself:** Expressing your gratitude out loud shows your partner that you appreciate and value what they do. This can help strengthen the emotional connection between you. But remember to be honest.

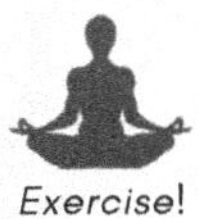

Exercise!

"Life will give you more than you're grateful for."

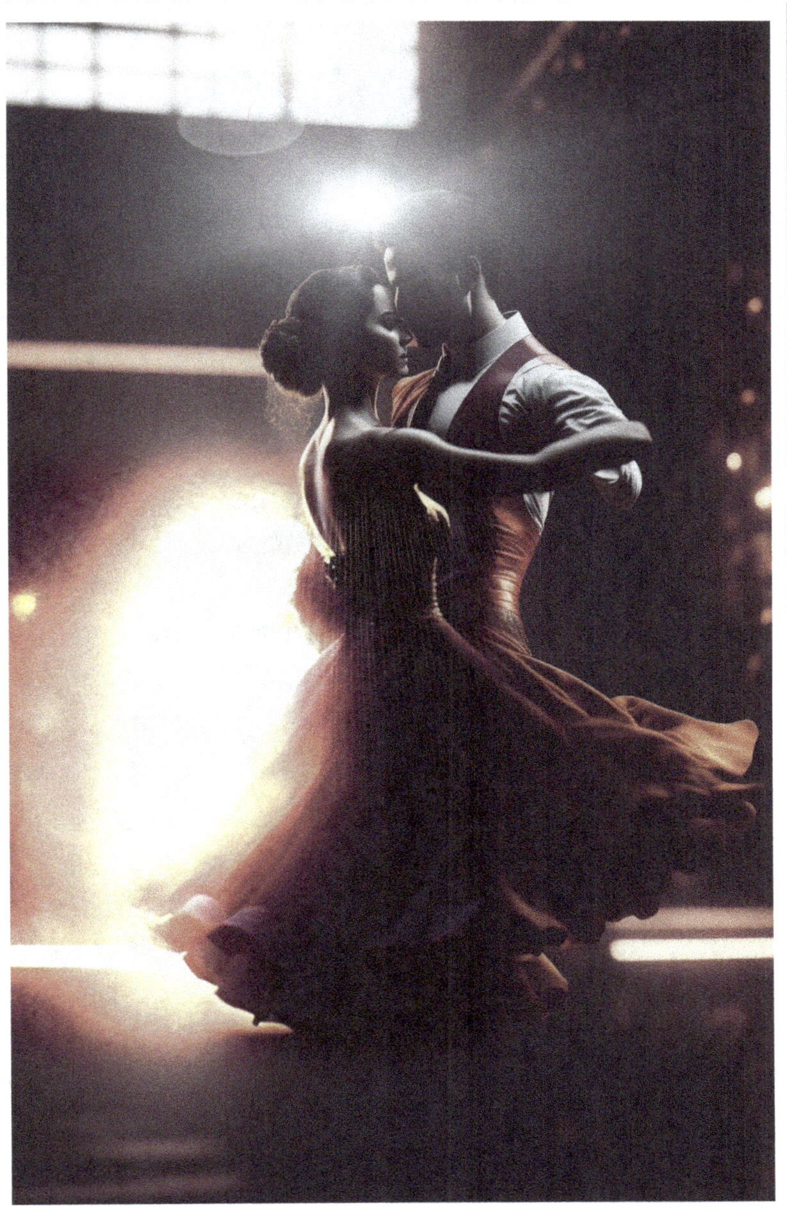

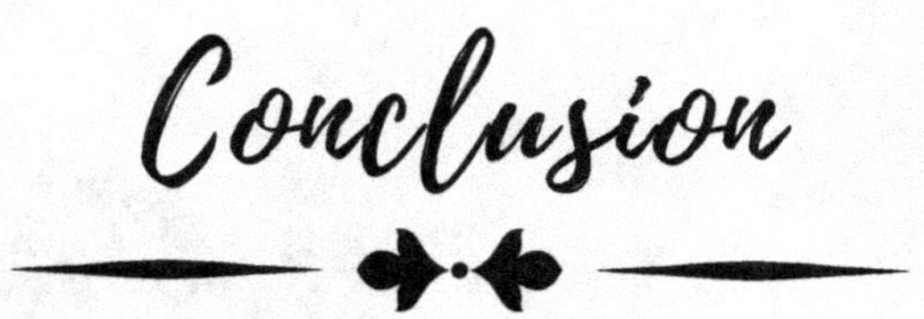

Conclusion

In this book, we provide practical tips and exercises to help you develop emotional and psychological skills to achieve a healthy marriage.

Remember that every relationship is unique and requires dedication and patience. Developing self-knowledge, communication, empathy, emotional intelligence, self-esteem, conflict resolution, forgiveness, gratitude, dealing with differences, dealing with expectations, dealing with routine, and maintaining passion are fundamental skills to build a lasting and meaningful relationship.

We hope this e-book has been helpful to you and we wish you success on your journey of personal development and healthy relationships.

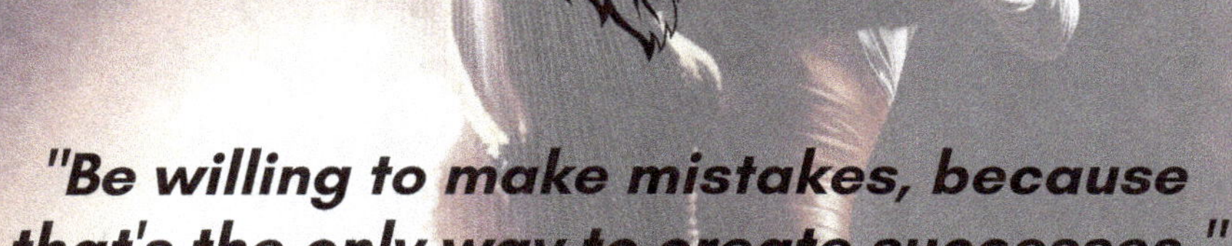

"Be willing to make mistakes, because that's the only way to create successes."

Nader El-Khouri

Entrepreneur, Business Administrator,
Family Father and **Living a Healthy Marriage**

Teresopolis - Rio de Janeiro - Brazil - 2023

Definitive Guide to Achieving a Healthy Marriage

www.ingramcontent.com/pod-product-compliance
Lightning Source LLC
Chambersburg PA
CBHW051652250726
48653CB00007B/2627